YOUR KNOWLEDGE HAS VALUE

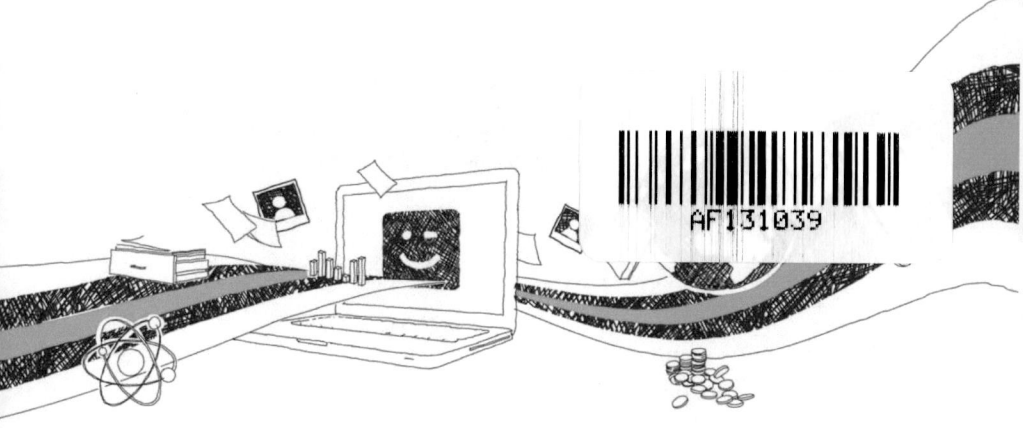

- We will publish your bachelor's and
  master's thesis, essays and papers

- Your own eBook and book -
  sold worldwide in all relevant shops

- Earn money with each sale

Upload your text at www.GRIN.com
and publish for free

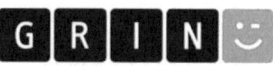

Bibliographic information published by the German National Library:

The German National Library lists this publication in the National Bibliography;
detailed bibliographic data are available on the Internet at http://dnb.dnb.de .

This book is copyright material and must not be copied, reproduced, transferred,
distributed, leased, licensed or publicly performed or used in any way except as
specifically permitted in writing by the publishers, as allowed under the terms and
conditions under which it was purchased or as strictly permitted by applicable
copyright law. Any unauthorized distribution or use of this text may be a direct
infringement of the author s and publisher s rights and those responsible may be
liable in law accordingly.

Imprint:

Copyright © 2012 GRIN Verlag, Open Publishing GmbH
Print and binding: Books on Demand GmbH, Norderstedt Germany
ISBN: 978-3-668-10057-2

This book at GRIN:

http://www.grin.com/en/e-book/311294/ayurveda-an-ancient-medical-system

Max Ande

Ayurveda. An ancient medical system

GRIN Publishing

GRIN - Your knowledge has value

Since its foundation in 1998, GRIN has specialized in publishing academic texts by students, college teachers and other academics as e-book and printed book. The website www.grin.com is an ideal platform for presenting term papers, final papers, scientific essays, dissertations and specialist books.

Visit us on the internet:

http://www.grin.com/

http://www.facebook.com/grincom

http://www.twitter.com/grin_com

Seminar paper on the topic of

Ayurveda

Student:	Maximilian Claudio Ande
Degree course:	KOM
Semester:	1st

Declaration on: 14.03.2012

Content

1. Introduction

If people living in the western civilization think about medicine the first thoughts coming to their minds may be medical scrubs, syringes, illness, science and a lot of complicated words they don't understand. Terms like philosophy, prevention, responsibility and being in tune with one's self and the environment aren't directly related to the orthodox medicine. But that's what Ayurveda, mankind's oldest medical system, is all about. Ayurveda is the doctrine of longevity, it's a religious based science of how to live one's daily life. This over 3000 years old scheme, invented by wise men who got together at the foot of the Himalaya Mountains looking for methods to cure diseases, recognizes a close relationship between human and a universe where everything (plants, rocks, animals) is inspired.

On the following pages I will look at Ayurvedic medicine, with its basic assumptions, most important forms of therapy, remedies and its special nutrition system.[1]

2. Ayurveda: A millenium-old concept of life

2.1. The Basics of Ayurveda medicine

The Vedas composed by the Rhesis at the foot of the Himalaya form the basics of Ayurvedic medicine. They include the first thesis about diagnosis, therapy and measures of sanitation. The Vedas are apaurusheya; an uncreated, timeless, unmanifested reality.[2] This means they are subject to constant change, which makes adding of different Sanskrits (medical writings on palm leaves) by different Weidjas (that's how ayurvedic doctors are called) possible. This adding of new knowledge allowed Ayurveda to improve itself over thousands of years.[3]

The three most important extensions of the Vedas are: The Caraka Samhita, which unites philosophy with anthropological medical facts, the Sushruta Samhita, where particular attention is given to surgery, which was nearly forgotten after the Buddhist influence on India in the year 300 before Christ, and the Ashtanga Hridaya Samhita, which is a flatly classification of Ayurvedic medicine in eight categories:

Kaya Cikitsa (Internal medicine), Bala Cikitsa (Pediatrics), Graha Cikitsa (Psychiatry), Shalya (Surgery), Shalakya Tantra (Ophthalmology, otolaryngology), Agada Tantra

---

[1] (Lad 13-18)

[2] (Schrott 10)

[3] (The Moving Visuals Co., narrator)

(toxicology), Rasayana Tantra (longevity and rejuvenation), Vajikarana Tantra (Eugenics and aphrodisiacs).[4], [5], [6]

2.2. The three Doshas

In the ayurvedic science, every human consists of a distinct composition of the five elements fire, water, air, terra and ether. These five elements appear in the human body as three bioenergetics, the Doshas: Vata, Pitta and Kapha, which control all body functions as holistic concepts. The percentage amount of every Dosha is determined at the fertilization and is termed as Prakriti. As a result, one, two, or all Doshas can exist in one human, whereby the dominating Dosha characterizes the physical and mental tees. That principle results in seven different constitutional types: Vata, Pitta, Kapha, Vata-Pitta, Pitta-Kapha, Vata-Kapha, Vata-Pitta-Kapha. In the further course the three Doshas will be explained.

Vata: Is composed of the elements ether and air. It stands for movement and flow. Vata steers movements in the body like breathing, muscle movement or fluctuation of the cytoplasm. It's the pacesetter of biological action and controls Pitta and Kapha. Humans with a dominant Vata-Dosha, are slender build and got a lot of energy. Their mind is active and restless.

Pitta: Pitta means fire and consists of the elements fire and water, whereby fire dominates. Pitta steers metabolism, digestion and even understanding and intelligence. People with a dominating Pitta-Dosha are normal build. They got a high intelligence and tend to be aggressive.

Kapha: Kapha means biological water and consists of the elements water and terra. It's the Dosha that gives structure to the body. It forms bones, muscles, sinews and all other tissue types. In addition, it is also responsible for the proper function of the immune system. People with a dominating Kapha-Dosha tend to obesity. They are slow and smoothly (physically and mental).

According to the three Doshas, there are three Gunas. Sattwa represents understanding, purity, clarity, compassion and love. Rajas embodies movement, aggression and

---

[4] (Schrott 10-16)

[5] (The Moving Visuals Co., narrator)

[6] (Pandora Film, Dr. B. G. Gokulan)

extraversion. And last but not least Tamas, which displays nescience, lethargy and stupor.[7]

2.3. The Dhatus and Srotas

In the Ayurveda, there are 7 different tissue types, the Dhatus. The Dhatus are chronologically related elements, which give the body structure and ensure the proper function of all organs. If one Dhatu fails, it will affect the following Dhatu. The chronology of the Dhatus is constructed as seen below.

1. Rasa (plasma): Contains nutrients of the digested food and provides all organs, tissue types and body systems.
2. Rakta (blood): Manages the oxidation in all tissue types and organs. Preserves one's life.
3. Mamsa (muscle): Protects the sensitive, vital organs. Manages the movement of joints. Keeps the physical strength of the body working.
4. Meda (fat): Makes everything greasy, makes the tissue types lubricated.
5. Asthi (bones): Stabilizes the body structure.
6. Majja (bone marrow and nerves): Fills the bones and mediates motoric and sensory impulses.
7. Shukra and Artav (Genitals): Consists of all tissue types and makes propagation possible.[8]

The ayurvedic medicine assumes canal systems existing throughout the human body, the Srotas. There are providing Srotas like the bronchial tubes or the gastrointestinal system and Srotas managing the transport of waste products like the urinary passages or the colon. Even lymph and capillary are Srotas.[9]

For a better understanding of the ayurvedic medicine I'd like to add, that the fire of the digestion is called Agni. Agni helps keeping the immune system in shape. Additionally the body produces three juices, the Malas (fecal, urine and sweat).[10]

Ayurveda is, like you see, very comprehensive, that's why there would be much more things to explain. That would however go beyond the scope of this paper, so I won't explain further details concerning basics of Ayurveda. The knowledge given on the first pages is enough to understand the information on the following sides.

---

[7] (Lad 19-31)

[8] (Lad 39-41)

[9] (Ranade 84-85)

[10] (Lad 35-38)

3. Ayurvedic therapy

3.1. Health and illness

The Sushruta Samhita says, that human is salutary, once:

-he's got a balanced physiology.

-his digestion and metabolism works well.

-the tissues and excretion are within the normal range.

-the soul is in a stage of happiness.

The process of getting sick, can be explained in a very simple way. The Doshas can get unbalanced by harmful influences like wrong nutrition, climate, seasons, life style or bad feelings. This leads to a weakness of Agni, what anon makes Ama (undigested nurture and toxics) appear. Ama now accumulates in the human body and clogs the Srotas. Toxic residues will gather at the weak spots of the body, where then diseases manifest.[11]

Now the aim is to get the Doshas back into balance by activating the self-healing power of the body. The emerged chaos in case of the disease needs to get organized again. A skilled person, who knows his body well, is able to recognize an imbalance of his Doshas at an early stage. He can react immediately by changing his life style and nutrition the right way. At this point it can be obviously seen, that one of the basics of Ayurveda is the science of one's daily life.[12]

3.2. Diagnoses and therapy

When it comes to healing in Ayurveda, Vaidyas are open-minded in concern of other medical influences, like for example the allopathic medicine. For example the guru Brahmanand Swamigal thinks, that the best aspects of the western medicine and Ayurvedic medicine should be combined in order to get the best results.[13]

Ayurvedic doctors don't do scans or screenings, because they aren't looking for a special disease, they recognize the human as a whole system, which is searched for imbalances. The first thing, vaidyas are doing, is to check the Doshas for imbalances. When there are previous scans from allopathic doctors, they certainly include them in their diagnose process.[14], [15]

---

[11] (Frawley 77-83)

[12] (Lad 33)

[13] (Pandora Film, Brahmanand Swamigal)

[14] (The Moving Visuals Co., narrator)

[15] (The Moving Visuals, Dr. Nandalal, Dr. Ragu)

To examine the balance of the Doshas, they take a look at the eyes, the tongue, the finger nails, the lips and the Nadhi (the pulse). This way they can determine which Dosha got out of balance. [16]

The definition of the disease is not being made before this investigation. Thereby possible sources of the disease get inquired in close collaboration with the patient. Afterwards, the stage of the disease gets ascertained. Vaidyas try to spot a disease as soon as possible, so that they can get a treatment success by just slightly changing the life style and nutrition of the patient or by perscribing safe herbs and minerals. [17], [18]

In general, the most important thing to notice is, that a vaidya doesn't treat diseases, he treats humans, what makes a positive relationship between doctor and patient essential. Such a positive relationship is the first step towards recovery, because it leads to happiness, which is one of the terms defining health. [19]

3.3. Pancha Karma

Once a serious illness has materialized itself that can't be cured by simply changing the daily life, or in case of chronic diseases, the patient is getting treated with Pancha Karma. Pancha Karma is a purification procedure during which the body gets rid of harmful residues. The meaning of Pancha Karma is to execute five different actions at the same time. These five actions are Vaman (vomiting), Virechan (use of laxative), Basti (enemas) and Nasya (introducing medicine through the nose). In phase one, the Doshas are being activated by giving the patient Ghee (a butter-herb mixture). After that, the patient gets a massage with herbal oils, to extract the residues out of the body. Thereupon vomiting, enemas and the introduction of oil through the nose is leading the toxics out of the body. Afterwards, body, mind and Doshas get closed by letting the patient take relaxing flower baths combined with steam bath sojourns. A treatment like this can be done stationary or ambulant and needs to be done for about two weeks, to get significant results. [20], [21]

---

[16] (Pandora Film, Brahmanand Swamigal)

[17] (Schrott 33-37)

[18] (meine-gesundheit)

[19] (Pandora Film, Brahmanand Swamigal)

[20] (Lad 64-65)

[21] (Schrott 35-42)

4. Medicinal substances

In the past, the ayurvedic knowledge only got passed on from Guru to scholar and the veidya got visited by his patients in his small surgery. In addition to the traditional veidyas, there are nowadays academically qualified Ayurveda doctors, who studied Ayurvedic medicine at a university, working in huge Ayurveda hospitals, like the Area Vaidya hospital in Katakal. In this type of hospitals, which can be found in every bigger city in India or Sri Lanka, patients only get treated with ayurvedic therapies and the special ayurvedic healing preparations.[22], [23]

All healing preparations used in the Ayurvedic medicine, are natural products, because human and nature are related to each other, meaning that health for the society, health for the human and health for the nature are all the same.[24]

In case of the preparation of Ayurvedic medicine, the effect of the herbs and minerals is as important as their taste. The preparations are taken in form of Chumas (powder), Kalkas (paste), Gutis (pills), jelly, herb wine and Tailas (oils). Most of the preparations are taken with Anupanams (medium of transport), like honey, sugar, coffee, milk or ghee, which reinforce the effect of the medicine.[25], [26]

5. Ayurvedic nutrition

Like already mentioned, nutrition has got a high priority in the Ayurveda, because the Doshas can inter alia get influenced through the food intake.[27]

The alimentation should be well-balanced, full-fledged and adjusted to a certain age, occupation and the dominating Dosha. In the Ahara (the ayurvedic dietetics), the senses smell, taste and the sight of the food get particular attention. The senses communicate with the internal needs, which are related to the Doshas, which in turn tell the human whether an aliment is good or bad for him.

In general, there are six different flavors, which got different features. Bitter (purging and stimulates liver and gall), sweet (stimulates the pancreas), sour (stimulates and boosts gastric glands and the production of saliva), salty (appetizing and sways the water supply), harsh (astringent and reassures the mucosa) and hot (stimulates metabolism, generates heat and scavenges the body).

---

[22] (Pandora Film, Brahmanand Swamigal)

[23] (The Moving Visuals Co., narrator)

[24] (Pandora Film, Dr. Nicolos Kostopoulos)

[25] (Schrott 37-40)

[26] (Frawley 412-413)

[27] (Schrott 66-69)

This way it is possible to create a special nutritional protocol for every constitution type under the consideration of the flavors, the Gunas (physical properties of food, like heavy, light, warm and cold) and the signs, which the Doshas give to the senses[28]

6. Conclusion

To conclude my paper, I want to present the current situation in terms of Ayurveda, taking a look at Germany and the United States of America. Referred to Germany, Ayurveda is getting more and more attention. Many hotels nowadays provide ayurvedic wellness treatments under the designation Maharishi Ayur Veda. Even though most attention is given to the relaxing factor, you can even find some surgeries providing the holistic range of Ayurveda treatment. It is also possible to study Ayurvedic medicine in Germany at the Rosenberg academy. The situation in North America is almost the same, where facilities like the American Institute of Vedic Science provide ayurvedic knowledge to the society. In general, Ayurveda is getting more attention in the western world from day to day. This is not at least attributable to the fact, that mankind's oldest science of life and medicine gives a solution to relive stress, the widespread disease of the western society, by teaching the people how to get in tune with oneself and mother nature.[29], [30], [31], [32]

---

[28] (Schacker 45-50)

[29] (ratgeber-blog)

[30] (augustayurveda, Dr. Sanjay Parva)

[31] (Rosenberg Akademie)

[32] (Pandora Film, Dr. Scott Gerson)

7. References

1: Lad, Vasant. Das große Ayurveda – Heilbuch: Die umfassende Einführung in das Ayurveda. Mit praktischen Anleitungen zur Selbstdiagnose, Therapie und Heilung. Aitrang: Windpferd Verlagsgesellschaft mbH, 1988.

2: Schrott, Ernst. Ayurveda für jeden Tag. Munich: Mosaik Verlag GmbH, 1994.

3: the Moving Visuals Co. Producers: Khim Loh, Galen Yeo. Directors: Christine Lim, Galen Yeo. Ayurveda – Indiens Weg des Heilens, 2002.

4: Schrott, Ernst. Ayurveda für jeden Tag. Munich: Mosaik Verlag GmbH, 1994.

5: the Moving Visuals Co. Producers: Khim Loh, Galen Yeo. Directors: Christine Lim, Galen Yeo. Ayurveda – Indiens Weg des Heilens, 2002.

6: Pandora Film, Sunrise Film & Pandora Medien, Monsoon Films, Filmbüro NW. Ayurveda – Art of being. 2001.

7: Lad, Vasant. Das große Ayurveda – Heilbuch: Die umfassende Einführung in das Ayurveda. Mit praktischen Anleitungen zur Selbstdiagnose, Therapie und Heilung. Aitrang: Windpferd Verlagsgesellschaft mbH, 1988.

8: Lad, Vasant. Das große Ayurveda – Heilbuch: Die umfassende Einführung in das Ayurveda. Mit praktischen Anleitungen zur Selbstdiagnose, Therapie und Heilung. Aitrang: Windpferd Verlagsgesellschaft mbH, 1988.

9: Ranade, Subhash. Ayurveda – Wesen und Methodik. Stuttgart: Haug Verlag, 1994.

10: Lad, Vasant. Das große Ayurveda – Heilbuch: Die umfassende Einführung in das Ayurveda. Mit praktischen Anleitungen zur Selbstdiagnose, Therapie und Heilung. Aitrang: Windpferd Verlagsgesellschaft mbH, 1988.

11: Frawley, David. Das große Ayurveda – Heilungsbuch, Prinzipien und Praxis. München: Droemersche Verlagsanstalt, 1999.

12: Lad, Vasant. Das große Ayurveda – Heilbuch: Die umfassende Einführung in das Ayurveda. Mit praktischen Anleitungen zur Selbstdiagnose, Therapie und Heilung. Aitrang: Windpferd Verlagsgesellschaft mbH, 1988.

13: Pandora Film, Sunrise Film & Pandora Medien, Monsoon Films, Filmbüro NW. Ayurveda – Art of being. 2001.

14: the Moving Visuals Co. Producers: Khim Loh, Galen Yeo. Directors: Christine Lim, Galen Yeo. Ayurveda – Indiens Weg des Heilens, 2002.

15: the Moving Visuals Co. Producers: Khim Loh, Galen Yeo. Directors: Christine Lim, Galen Yeo. Ayurveda – Indiens Weg des Heilens, 2002.

16: Pandora Film, Sunrise Film & Pandora Medien, Monsoon Films, Filmbüro NW. Ayurveda – Art of being. 2001.

17: Schrott, Ernst. Ayurveda für jeden Tag. Munich: Mosaik Verlag GmbH, 1994.

18: "Medizin mal anders". http//www.meine-gesundheit.de/natur/texte/ . Date of access: 1.03.2012.

19: Pandora Film, Sunrise Film & Pandora Medien, Monsoon Films, Filmbüro NW. Ayurveda – Art of being. 2001.

20: Lad, Vasant. Das große Ayurveda – Heilbuch: Die umfassende Einführung in das Ayurveda. Mit praktischen Anleitungen zur Selbstdiagnose, Therapie und Heilung. Aitrang: Windpferd Verlagsgesellschaft mbH, 1988.

21: Schrott, Ernst. Gesund und jung mit Ayurveda – Die sanfte Heilweise für vollkommene Gesundheit und inneres Gleichgewicht. München: Mosaik Verlag GmbH, 1996.

22: Pandora Film, Sunrise Film & Pandora Medien, Monsoon Films, Filmbüro NW. Ayurveda – Art of being. 2001.

23: the Moving Visuals Co. Producers: Khim Loh, Galen Yeo. Directors: Christine Lim, Galen Yeo. Ayurveda – Indiens Weg des Heilens, 2002.

24: Pandora Film, Sunrise Film & Pandora Medien, Monsoon Films, Filmbüro NW. Ayurveda – Art of being. 2001.

25: Schrott, Ernst. Gesund und jung mit Ayurveda – Die sanfte Heilweise für vollkommene Gesundheit und inneres Gleichgewicht. München: Mosaik Verlag GmbH, 1996.

26: Frawley, David. Das große Ayurveda – Heilungsbuch, Prinzipien und Praxis. München: Droemersche Verlagsanstalt, 1999.

27: Schrott, Ernst. Ayurveda für jeden Tag. Munich: Mosaik Verlag GmbH, 1994.

28: Schacker, Reinhart. Das Ayurveda Lebensbuch – Ein praktischer Leitfaden für eine gesunde und bewusste Lebensführung. Amsterdam: Iris Bücher & mehr, 2000.

29: "fernöstliche Medizin - Ayurveda in Deutschland". Blog.de/tb/a/r/fernoestliche-medizin/ayurveda-in-deutschland/4464128/ . Date of access: 10.03.2012.

30: Dr. Sanjay Parva. "Ayurveda in America today". Augustayurveda.com/wellness1.asp?id=12 . Date of access: 10.03.2012.

31: Europäische Akademie für Ayurveda. www.ayurveda-akademie.org/home/ . Date of access: 10.03.2012.

32: Pandora Film, Sunrise Film & Pandora Medien, Monsoon Films, Filmbüro NW. Ayurveda – Art of being. 2001.

YOUR KNOWLEDGE HAS VALUE

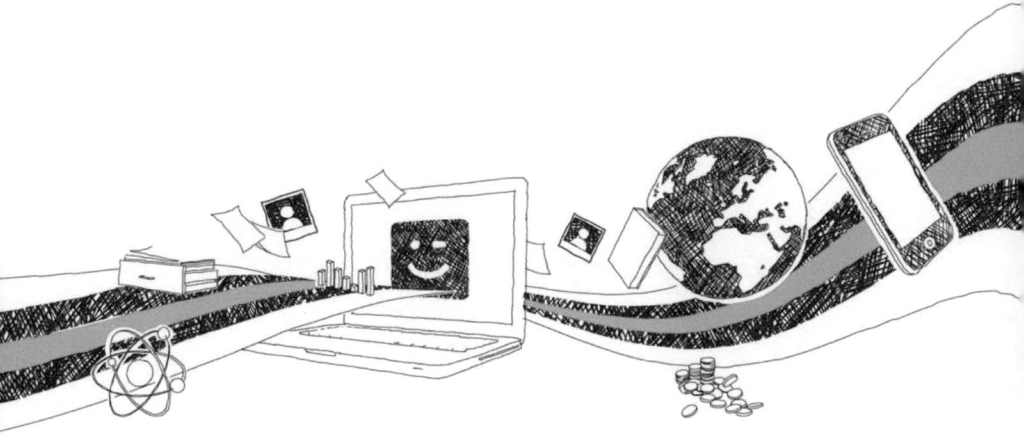

- We will publish your bachelor's and
  master's thesis, essays and papers

- Your own eBook and book -
  sold worldwide in all relevant shops

- Earn money with each sale

Upload your text at www.GRIN.com
and publish for free

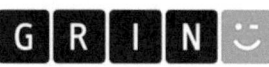